T0106130

MAN IS THE EXTENSION OF WOMAN

(Know the Ultimate Truth about Yourself)

DR. MAKARAND FULZELE

iUniverse, Inc.
Bloomington

Man Is the Extension of Woman
Know the Ultimate Truth about Yourself

iUniverse books may be ordered through booksellers or by contacting:

iUniverse
1663 Liberty Drive
Bloomington, IN 47403
www.iuniverse.com
1-800-Authors (1-800-288-4677)

*Because of the dynamic nature of the Internet, any web addresses or links
contained in this book may have changed since publication and may no longer be
valid. The views expressed in this work are solely those of the author and do not
necessarily reflect the views of the publisher, and the publisher hereby disclaims
any responsibility for them.*

*Any people depicted in stock imagery provided by Thinkstock are models,
and such images are being used for illustrative purposes only.*

Certain stock imagery © Thinkstock.

ISBN: 978-1-4759-4944-5 (sc)
ISBN: 978-1-4759-4945-2 (e)

Library of Congress Control Number: 2012916683

Printed in the United States of America

iUniverse rev. date: 12/6/2012

Devoted to the spirit of light!

Contents

Preface

Medical profession is noble and I am blessed to be a part of it. It is one of those rarest professions that take you very close to other people. You see life in its many forms. In a very special way medical science has opened my eyes to infinite possibilities. Some divine plan is already working inside the bodies of us all. That includes not only humankind but whole of living matter including microorganisms. There are some simple clues regarding what would be that divine plan.

As a doctor and more so as a surgeon, I regularly get to view inside of human body. I get to see thousands of such clues routinely. These signs are subtle but definitely present. I feel I have found one such simple yet profound link to the bigger plan. This book is all about that simple but hidden truth.

A few years back when I was studying *'anatomy'* for my medical training course, this thought crossed my mind for the first time. However I ignored it choosing to focus instead on more pressing matter of academics. I got busy in trying to know the things already known to science. The thought was buried deep inside. Occasionally on a dark and lonely day, it would raise its head. Nonetheless I was able to suppress it. Soon I became a surgeon, got married. Participating in the race of life, I had totally forgotten about the thought. Meanwhile I had already written a book titled *'Rainbow'*.

'Rainbow' was my first attempt at writing. It was published by iUniverse. By then I had settled in life. That is when this thought again cropped up. It refused to leave me. It used to make me restless. If I tried to dump it, it would agitate my mind. At times, it consumed me. It demanded my total unwavering attention. At more susceptible times when I was free, it would create lot of turbulence and shake me up. At one such weaker moment, I decided to capture it. This book is my sincere effort to pass on this turbulence to receptive minds.

I am not a feminist. I don't claim to have achieved a scientific milestone. I don't deal with subject of life after death. And I don't want to sound like a philosophical Guru.

No doubt, this book would appeal to the open and impartial mind. Open your eyes to see what I have seen and you would be thrilled to grasp the small reality about us.

What is the difference between man and woman? The answer is obvious, isn't it? Or just wait a moment. What if the answer is not so obvious? What if the truth is different than what we have perceived so far?

Existing knowledge about man and woman has failed to answer many questions. Man, for example, has struggled to understand woman and woman has not been able to make the man adopt her way of thinking.

We think that man and woman are poles apart. It is very deeply ingrained in our minds. There are even books like, *'Men are from Mars and Women are from Venus'*. Though I have not gone through the book, the title gives the message that man and woman are different.

Sands of time have passed over the stories of Adam and Eve. They are no more in the jungles. Man has conquered the moon. Woman has followed suit travelling in 'discovery'. We now live in modern age. Woman is working side by side with man in every sphere of life. Mindset of a man has changed too. But even today in different parts of globe, man and woman are not considered equal.

Like many, I am also a product of similar society. It told us woman is delicate and man is strong by nature, hence man should protect her and she should serve him in return. Social norms dictate the behavior of a woman. Many such differences were imprinted on my mind. Even the God had said that man would be master of woman. She would have to undergo labor pains and bear his children. The more interesting story is one in which Eve was created from the rib of Adam.

Course in medicine changed my thinking style. Everything, every belief had to have a reason otherwise it was discarded. It was kind of evolution of mind that transplanted new ideas in the place of non-working archaic ideas. In a different environment, I put old theory under the microscope of medical knowledge. What I saw was entirely different than my previous perception. The mind had awakened to another possibility. I just could not discard this thought, this new idea as an illusion of mind.

Sunlight is the best disinfectant. Test your belief in the new light. You may or may not agree with me. Your world will not change if you do not agree with me. But if you agree with me, how does it change your world? If more people agree with you and me, how does it change our world? The possibilities are limitless.

Namaste-

Dr. Makarand Fulzele

Mumbai (India)

Introduction

Man and woman are different. They look different. They sound different. They think differently. No doubt, man is different than woman. Psychologically, physically and behavior wise they are different. The base of all living matter is genes. Man and woman are different genetically too! We have dwelt upon these facts for twenty one centuries or even more.

But what seems different at first sight may not be different at all. There is a famous story about Birbal, a clever man working for Akbar, the great Mughal Emperor. Birbal was once asked by the emperor the difference between truth and lie. The great Birbal answered "just four fingers". He was clearly referring to the distance between eyes and ears. What he meant was, what we hear is not complete truth unless and until we have seen it with our eyes.

Today we are aware that what we see with our eyes may not be the complete truth. The visual sensation can be an illusion. Vision is nothing but the perception of the brain created by the illusion of the light. As the content of the light changes so does the perception. Illusions can be created or are inborn errors of the brain. A man can see a rope as snake in the darkness of night. Certain drugs can make you see things differently than they really are. Entire world of magicians is based upon this one principle. This topic is endless and it is fruitless to go deeper into it. Moreover, it would divert our attention from subject under consideration. Just understand here that eye is not the absolute judge of the truth. What appears …… may not be. So men and women obviously appear to be different, but are they? They are not.

They are not different emotionally, intellectually and least physically, though it may appear so. Behavior wise they are very different as they consider themselves different from each other, based upon above criteria. This difference too may disappear once they consider each other equal.

I have already said that men and women are similar. But that's not all I want to say. All philosophers including Vivekananda, the famous Yogi, have described human life as a path which does not end with death. Putting philosophy aside and bringing in the science, I say the same thing. Human life is a common pathway on which man and woman are travelling in same direction. Only difference is that, man is little bit ahead of a woman on the same path. They are at different points. Nonetheless man was at the same point where woman is now and if woman continues to travel she will reach the point where man is at present.

To make it simple, forget the road. Consider a staircase with ten steps. If third step represents the womanhood then man is probably at fourth or even fifth step.

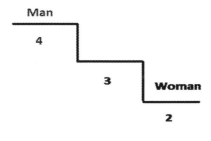

Staircase of Evolution

But how has he reached the fourth step? He has not bypassed the previous steps. He has gone step by step to reach fourth step.

With this preamble, let us move forward. A slow and gradual introduction will develop the concept.

As a doctor I had access to certain knowledge which other people might not have. This knowledge has undergone a critical dissection inside my mind to arrive at certain inferences. My aim is to put it in front of the world. I don't claim to have reached a breakthrough in human science. It is the restlessness inside that is vented outside.

To take us to our destination, we will state certain hypothetical things which are not proven yet. This is essential as I, the writer, don't have means to prove them. The people who have means may not be interested in proving them simply because thought of looking at prevalent evidence in a different way may not have occurred to them.

At this stage, I am going to make two statements which are interconnected.

- Man has to go through a stage of womanhood before he achieves his masculinity

- If a woman lives long enough she will be converted into a man

My childhood hero was Sherlock Holmes. In fact my teacher always used to say, a shrewd clinician should be like Sherlock Holmes. On one occasion, Mr. Holmes tells Dr. Watson, "People consider me brilliant because I directly tell the inference. People are shocked and think that I am some sort of genius. But if I start telling them how in step by step manner I have reached the conclusion, they will lose interest. In fact they might consider it ordinary".

Knowingly or unknowingly I have followed my hero and put the conclusion first. Right away, it may sound difficult to digest. Let your mind ruminate these statements.

In the meanwhile, let us revisit the differences between man and woman. For simplification, they are divided into five categories:

- Genetic

- Anatomical

- Intellectual

- Psychological (emotional)

- Behavior patterns

We will discuss these differences in detail and we will realize that ultimately there is no difference at all. We will awaken to the possibility of man and woman being part of the same process in different time zones.

We look at things and accept them according to our beliefs. Two people could look at the same thing and arrive at diametrically opposite conclusions. Stories and exercises on perceptions abound in corporate world. If you search for 'optical illusions' on the net, you will come across many images that would confuse the mind as it tries to come to grip with reality and perceived reality.

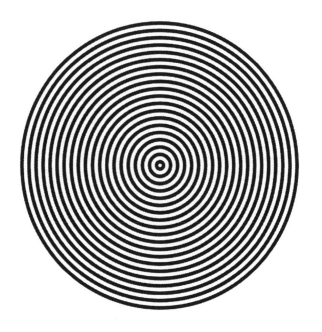

The above image illustrates the point I want to make. We know for sure that the circles aren't moving but if we focus on the innermost circle and if our gaze lingers there for a while then it gives us a feeling of a vortex.

Once we learn that man and woman are not different and the perceived reality about differences between them is not real then it would make us wonder, how could we ignore it for so long?

PART-I
It's All about Genetics

Basic Things First...........

We will discuss simple genetic aspect with regard to our hypothesis.

Let's concentrate upon fundamental factors. Twenty three pairs of chromosomes exist amongst us all. Many of you may know this already. But knowing this is not enough. Analyzing and applying it to reach a particular inference, is important.

Twenty three pairs of chromosomes are present in all of us out of which twenty two pairs are autosomes which are similar in both man and woman. That's right. Out of twenty-three pairs, twenty-two pairs are similar irrespective of gender. Don't be surprised. Instead let us focus on what it could mean for the mankind. If these autosomes are similar then they should lead to similar results in man as well as woman, isn't it? Correct! These autosomes are mainly concerned with development of human body that's common in both - man and woman. They contribute similar development in man and woman and none of these autosomes can make a woman different from a man.

In general, genes are like a blueprint based on which the human body is constructed. But as I have discussed above, as far as our theme is concerned we no longer need these twenty two pairs of autosomes which are same in both sexes. These twenty-two pairs help us to understand basic similarity between man and woman. To move to the next level, we will need to direct our attention to the 23rd pair of chromosomes. It is the most important player in our analysis.

The twenty third pair is called sex chromosomes. This is at the root of all differences between man and woman.

- The pair of sex chromosomes in man is called X and Y

- The counterpart in woman is called X and X

Let us for a moment go away from our core subject. However, let me assure you that it is a short cut to take us to our goal rather quickly. Now I discuss what I call a 'two shirts theory'.

Two Shirts Theory

Man lived in a jungle for a long time. There were no clothes then. Over centuries, cotton was discovered and soon afterwards mankind learned to weave clothes. A great improviser came along and he stitched shirts. That era was known as era of shirts. After designing variety of beautiful shirts, the tailor of the shirts got tired and decided to take a nap.

One man living in an era of shirts went to a shop and bought two shirts. In the process he exhausted his limited money. Another man went and bought just one shirt. He wanted to spare extra cash for future.

Time passed by. The world progressed. Our great improviser woke up from his rather long slumber. This time, he came up with another brilliant idea and designed a trouser. Remember, the gap between arrival of shirt and trouser was quite big.

The first man looks at the progress and sighs! He does not have enough money to buy the trousers. But the other guy goes and buys a trouser too. Their actions create a disparity. At any given moment the first man can use only one shirt while the other man wears a shirt as well as a pant.

From the point of utility, at any given time, the first man is effectively half naked. On the contrary, the smart guy is fully clothed.

For the first man it is like having an extra backup shirt. To improve utility, he can use both the shirts simultaneously. But it won't be much different from using one shirt at a time. It won't give him any added advantage. At all times he will be half naked.

Look at the smart guy. He is smartly dressed. He can step out any time to mix with any crowd. In that sense, he is more matured. He is more advanced. But do you think the two men are drastically different?

Imagine that the first man looks at the smart guy and decides something has to be done. He wants to bridge the gap between them. He reconsiders his situation and sacrifices his backup shirt. He somehow re-stitches it into a trouser to complete his wardrobe. At the same time, the smart guy goofs up, behaves carelessly and gets a hole in his trouser. These things can happen in the phenomenon called life.

Here is an analogy. The shirt is like 'X' chromosome and trouser is like 'Y' chromosome.

Man has X and Y chromosomes and woman has X and X chromosomes. X chromosomes are exactly similar which means woman is effectively only X chromosome. Mankind does not yet know the relevance of an extra X in woman. On the contrary, the extra X is known to have harmful effects of genetic disorders getting manifested in vulnerable woman. May be other X is acting as back up copy. However, the extra X does not play any role throughout the life of a woman.

Just remember, woman is only 'X' chromosome.

Compare woman with a man. He is something more. He is X and Y which implies he is essentially an 'X 'plus something extra. What do I mean by that? Man is already a woman that is 'X', plus something extra. Does that mean first step towards manhood is womanhood?

Let's use some basic mathematics. Here is the equation,

Man $= 22$ autosomes $+ X + Y$

Woman $= 22$ autosomes $+ X + X$

$= 22$ autosomes $+ X$ (by logic not by mathematics

$\therefore$ Man $= (22$ autosomes $+ X) + Y$

$=$ Woman $+ Y$

Thus man is everything that woman is, plus something extra. This extra thing is not qualitatively different, but quantitatively.

Hence Y here must be somewhat like X + 1, X+2 or X+ 3 or something like that.

Whoever has named the chromosomes x and y, must have named them by instinct. May be he had same thing in mind as I have. Did he go through the same thought process that I am taking you through? Did he realize that the man is the extension of woman or in other words the man had to go through a process of becoming a woman? Because the points discussed above -

Woman = 22 autosomes + X + X

= 22 autosomes + X (by logic not by mathematics)

∴ Man = (22 autosomes + X) + Y

= Woman + Y

- are indirectly implied by giving Woman chromosome a name of X chromosome and Man chromosome a name of Y chromosome. As Y comes after X in English alphabet similarly a Man comes after Woman.

I repeat, the person who named chromosomes as X and Y must have gone through the same understanding that I am bringing to your attention – 'Man is the extension of Woman'.

It would be ultimately proven that woman can potentially grow into a man. Similarly man can reduce to a woman, if he loses some part of 'Y'.

At deeper level, my thoughts about genetics have always projected them as a blue print. Our bodies are structures build upon this blue print. Nature can use only twenty two autosomes plus X and Y, to lay the foundation.

Genetics need to be explained a bit more. They are the basic support on which the whole building of human body gets built.

In the womb of a woman, lying quietly or sometimes kicking or trying to swim, in the sea of the amniotic fluid (that is the fluid inside the amniotic sac covering the fetus) a future man or woman is lying without any distinction of sex. By that I mean both are similar. May I go further and add that both are females until certain stage. This stage is prominent function of the 'X' chromosome.

Body is like a shapeless stone and an artist called 'X' shapes it as a woman. Thereafter, slowly 'Y' too develops an interest in sculpting. He takes over as he is dominant by nature. 'Y' can't change what's already happened. But he can do something special. He adds some characters and suppresses some other characters.

In simple words,

Male and female are same in the beginning

Then they simultaneously develop into a female

- The 'X' stops here and a lady remains a lady

- But 'Y' pulls himself further into a male

In this blueprint, is there someone creating or suggesting that who will be male or otherwise? For believers, its god! For nonbelievers, its nature! Nature or God erase 'X' from same blueprint to replace it with 'Y'.

In humans the above said statement is not correct. Still I said it. In humans 'X' is not erased and replaced by 'Y'. But 'Y' is directly transferred from the male.

But do you know, how gender is decided in certain other beautiful people? The people with long tails, beautiful creased skins and big teeth? I am talking about alligators. Can you guess looking at them, who is male and who is not? Not unless you turn them upside down. You might come to know their gender but we may never know it from you.

Alligators don't have separate codes of behavior for male and female. They are both violent; they crush and play with their food. After the meal, they go and lie on the rocks in the Sun.

These alligators are going to provide us the clues we need.

To begin with, female alligator lays an egg. The genetic material is exactly the same in all eggs. Basically all eggs are to give birth to a female alligator. It has been observed that eggs will deliver males only if environmental heat is high. The heat changes the genetic blueprint to convert a female to a male. If environment is cold, female remains female. That was one of the most interesting knowledge shared on Discovery Channel.

This leads us to an exciting hypothesis. Consider the genetic difference in alligator male and female. It is just like man and woman. X and Y determine the gender of the animal. Above discussion proves that with heat 'X' can be converted into 'Y'. Does that mean 'Y' is liquefied "X"? Or do some connections inside Y melt with heat and get lost forever?

Likewise can a woman be converted into a man and vice versa with the use of heat? This heat factor seems to work in embryonic stage of alligator. In adult alligators, it does not lead to any change.

There is no direct evidence among humans about such happening. However, an indirect hint exists which we shall discuss in elaborate manner. It is known as *hot furnace syndrome*. In this syndrome men continuously exposed to hot temperature are prone to infertility. The reason is the irreversible changes in the testicles of the man due to heat. At continuously high temperatures, the testicles kind of disintegrate and are not able to function as primary reproductive organs. It is strange but true. The man loses his masculinity when exposed to persistent heat.

What does it lead us to?

Have you heard of *Chinese calendar of sex?* According to this calendar, a human pair of male and female can have sex at a particular time of the year and produce a child of desired gender. This calendar prescribes a period of the year for having sex if you want a boy and another period for a girl. This ensures a delivery at almost a particular period. We know that some seasons are cold, some are warm and some are hot. The pattern indicates that temperature plays a great role in determining sex of the human embryo.

Can we say, in the beginning we are all females? And that the heat decides who is going to be what?

Man and woman are not qualitatively different if we consider the genetics. The 'X' can be converted into 'Y'. The heat can make the necessary changes.

The title of this book is simple and innocuous. However, the contents are shocking and not so innocuous. It can lead to lot of confusion and disturb the image that we have created about our own self.

Let me highlight what I want to say:

- Till puberty man and woman are same

- If man lives longer, he can get converted into woman

- If woman lives longer, she can get matured into man

For a change, let us dive into the realm of stories.

Give me one second of your life. And in this second, do as I ask you! Just think that you have found the ultimate truth about life for which many yogis and saints are striving to reach.

Have you observed the life of great saints? Most of them have a similar life story. In the beginning they are rich and powerful. They live their life to fullest and they fight many wars. They have sex with beautiful women by will or by force. They drink the best wine and eat the best food. They enjoy the riches of life. The life for them is like an ever burning fire of desires. The vigor, the virility is the main feature.

As is to be expected, eventually they get bored and turn away from the path of evil. They become calm and peaceful, they start meditating. They then evolve to be great sages.

What exactly leads to change in their behavior? In the absence of scientific analysis, I use little bit of imagination here. As you would notice, the imagination may actually be true but mankind may have to wait for few years, decades or who knows centuries to arrive at it.

At the height of their wild ways, these rich and powerful people are using energy of the body at the maximum. This causes internal metabolism to boil. Testosterone, the male hormone flows abundantly. The internal metabolism produces heat, which causes 'Y' chromosome to melt and loose some part, to get converted into 'X'. These kings with the loss of 'Y' chromosome lose vital energy force; get evolved to sages – a stage that is more peaceful, non-aggressive and reasonable. The evolved characters are the characters that we associate mostly with the fairer sex. Continuing their journey, the meditation further opens their mind.

Only a soldier knows the value of peace! We all believe in that. It sounds very true when felt with our souls. But soldier understands it only after he has fought a terrible war not before it. This change of heart may also be due to the internal destruction of 'Y' leading to withering of aggression. There are many similar circumstances. I leave it to the esteemed reader to think deeply and find such situations. We may also look at our own life and observe how an old age brings about changes to our bodies that leave hardly any differences between man and woman.

Why would woman mature into man? Why would man get reduced to woman?

The answer lies in our genetic makeup. May be 'Y' loses some of its part in the long run and turns into 'X'. Similarly in woman, back up 'X' could get matured into 'Y'.

This genetic process till now is only in our minds or to be more accurate in my mind.

One should remember at this point that particular type of genetic material is the basis for the expression of the male or female bodies. Everything depends upon the blueprint of genetic map. Any change in the structure of male or female body if has to be brought, has to be brought up through the change in blueprint.

What alters these genes? I consider it to be hormones but about that we will talk much later. Till then we will discuss something different, the beautiful expression of the creator that has been designed by this genetic map – the human anatomy!

PART-II
The Beautiful Anatomy

Anatomical Differences between Man and Woman

Let's understand hypothesis that we have discussed so far. We have absorbed genetic blueprint concept. Having laid a blue print, let's see how this blue print expresses itself.

This manifestation though follows smooth, natural and systematic flow, it is very complex in nature. When I read embryological books, the process of actualization appeared so systematic and rhythmical that I thought the composer must be God. Unlike the popular perception, many times science helps to build your faith. Then you try to feel that invisible hand, behind everything.

The expression of genetic map is the beautiful human body. The body is beautiful as far as you don't go into details. However, it is inevitable for the further discussion of our topic. For simplification I have divided this discussion into two parts, external and internal.

External differences between woman and man are too obvious. They can be seen with naked eyes. Sometimes they are pleasant too. Here am I talking about Marilyn Monroe or what?

The internal differences are viewed in detail after dissection of the body. Sometimes we can use special scanning techniques like M.R.I or C.T. scans.

Let us now shift our focus to the external differences. Again we can divide them into two parts - sexual and nonsexual differences - to simplify the matters. Let's summarize this,

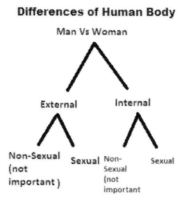

After much ado about nothing, we ultimately start with nonsexual differences. What are these? I will discuss the external and internal nonsexual differences together for simplification.

These are mainly differences in skin, hair, bones, muscles, nerves and the viscera. Viscera word as such contains the plethora of organs like heart, lungs, esophagus, intestines, stomach, liver and spleen. Then there is spinal cord in the spine and the brain.

Nerves and spinal cord are same in both. In men, the skeleton is bony. They have comparatively large muscle mass and less fat. Females are less bony, have less muscle and more fat.

Hair is the one thing, which differentiates the woman a lot from a man. Women have long hairs on scalp and men don't. But the hairs can be grown to length in males too. So it is just the matter of chance. But male have definite frontal regression on scalp. Males have more chance of going bald. Hair growth in axilla is similar, but females like to shave it off. Male have more body hair. They can grow hair on chest, considered for long to be a sign of masculinity. Women do have body hair but they love to shave it off. Pubic hair in male and female have different patterns.

In general, hair in man and woman are same except for the quantity and pattern.

These differences do not exist in heart, lung, liver, spleen or gastrointestinal tract except for the size. Size is matter of need of the body. That depends upon the life style and every day behavior patterns. Hormonal influence is also present, about which we will discuss much latter. As you can see, weight of these organs differ but the qualitative structure and function are same.

I have not discussed many other tissues in the body as it is not very important for our cause.

Important point to note here is that, the difference is only in quantity and arrangement not in the quality. So may I say as far as these nonsexual organs are concerned, man and woman are same?

To prove this point even further, in a pre-pubertal child, this difference is nonexistent. All the organs discussed above are same, even quantitatively in both the sexes. Then hormones come into play at puberty and they bring about the difference. Does that mean that not only in the womb of a mother, but even further till puberty when sexual differences make their appearance, man and woman are just the same?

Now let's move our discussion to sexual differences.

First we will discuss the external sexual differences. The breast is discussed separately.

Let's use some simple anatomical facts that we have at our disposal.

Let's start with vulva in females. Vulva is made of two lobes with cleft in between. The cleft opens outside and through this cleft vaginal and urethral orifices open to outside. It has got clitoris at the upper end of cleft. It looks like this:

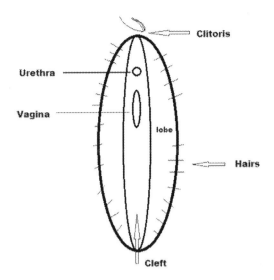

Clitoris has a role in sexual stimulation. In fact in some women, it is the most sensitive part. It also serves function of erection when sexually aroused.

Urethra or urethral opening is the external opening of the urinary tract. The kidney inside the body produces urine, which flows through ureter. Ureters are like pipelines. The two ureters from two kidneys open into one bladder. Bladder is nothing but a bag to store urine. Bladder through one urethra opens outside. Urinary expulsion is the function of urethral opening.

Vaginal opening located below the urethra inside vulval cleft is connected with uterus inside. Through this, semen goes inside the uterus. From here, through fallopian tubes, it goes up to its destination - the ovaries, where the zygote is formed.

So in simple words,

- Vulva is two lobes with cleft in between

- It contains vagina and urethra

- It has hair at the periphery

I sincerely hope that you have understood everything and that the anatomical knowledge is crystal clear in your mind.

Remember you are not yourself, but Steven Spielberg. So create a movie. Use imagination. Break your mind free. Imagine! Vulval cleft is disappearing and that it is getting fused from its lower end. What will happen?

Vagina and urethra starts shifting upward. It gets crowded at upper end, but the fusion still continues. Vagina and urethra are forced to fuse. The membrane separating vagina and urethra breaks down. As a result, there is only one opening, a common opening.

Fusion does not stop here. It pushes this common opening towards clitoris. Clitoris opens and engulfs this opening. In the process clitoral length increases and vulval fusion is over.

Imagine how it will look. Two lobes of the vulval fused with hair at periphery with clitoris enlarged containing the urethral and vaginal common opening.

Is it difficult to imagine?

It is a penis with common genitourinary opening, with scrotum with hair at periphery. Of course simultaneously some changes will be occurring inside of the body. I will discuss them, latter.

What are the equivalents?

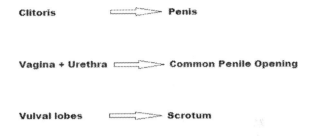

- Step one is clitoris at the top with two (vaginal and urethral) separate openings in the cleft of vulval folds.

- Step two is, penis with common urogenital opening and scrotum.

As far as external genitalia are concerned, woman is at step one. Whereas the man has already reached step two. So man is the extension of woman.

'X' chromosome forms female genitalia. 'Y' chromosome remains in hibernation. As soon as period of hibernation is over, 'Y' chromosome converts female genitalia into male genitalia. This obviously occurs in male. In female 'Y 'remains in hibernation over lifetime.

Is it difficult to digest? Don't worry. In one of the following chapters, I am going to discuss the differences between the internal genital organs of man and woman.

More clearly, how they are not different at all, except for the maturation level. This will clear all the doubts.

The female internal genital organs if matured will be converted into male genital organs.

In other words, basic blocks used for creation are same in male and female genital organs. The level of maturity and the complex arrangements are different. Man is more complex (contrary to popular belief).

Does that mean quality or even quantity of material used is same, except the patterning in male and female genitalia? Do you consider it, as a difference or gradation?

I think we are not different at all. Rather we are standing at the different points of the same road.

In the next chapter we will discuss the breasts!

Breasts

Breasts are prominent part of human body. As we look at them, it appears to be contrary to our conclusions.

A woman appears to be the extension of a man. It is the fault of the eye. For centuries we have depended too much on vision for understanding the truth. But visual perceptions don't tell the truth every time. I maintain that man is the extension of woman. The concept of breast development helps to prove it. How?

Woman is having larger breast with lot of fat and lactational glands that give it an attractive contour. Nipples are bigger.

In man, breasts are smaller with residual or no lactational glands and almost flat with no contour.

The smaller breasts in man and bigger development of breasts in woman might lead us to believe that woman should be an extension of man. It is time to find out the real truth. Let's go to the depth of the scenario.

'X' chromosome decides that the breast should be larger and bulky with lactational glands and longer nipples. But when does it occur? When does a girl become a woman with fully grown breasts?

Till puberty the breasts are similar in both the genders ……….. flat.

At puberty around twelve years of age in a female, a sudden large flow of hormonal secretions occurs. This brings about the above said changes. It is called *hormonal surge* in medical language. This surge is masterminded by 'X' chromosome. It is a Simple reaction of body to increased hormonal levels. What are these hormones is not important. Let's call them female hormones.

Remember that 'X' chromosome is also present in men. So this hormonal reaction should be seen in the men too, by analogy.

This is true except for the 'Y' chromosomal interferences that we are yet to discuss.

'X' and 'Y' chromosomes act in steps.

In short,

- Step I - flat chest

- Step II - female type of chest at puberty

There is a long period in between these two steps. Considering puberty occurs in females at around twelve years of age, so this period between step one and step two is more than a decade. The sleeping 'Y' chromosome awakens in males around the same time. However, the

'Y' chromosome decides to intervene before the step II. He takes the third step (discussed below) before the second step is manifested in males.

So what do we observe?

Step one and 'Y' chromosomal interference manifested as stagnation of step one in males. As both these steps are similar in males, they are not noticed separately.

So in summary the development of females and males is as follows:

	Female	**Male**
Step I	Flat chest	Flat chest
Step II	Female type of chest	Female type of chest suppressed by
		'Y' chromosome
		End result → flat chest

Thus we should not forget that 'Y' chromosome reverses the process even before it is started.

Do not be baffled by above claims. They may appear little bit farfetched at this juncture because I have not given you the evidences. Be patient. I will share with you relevant medical facts at the right time.

Have you ever heard the *phenomenon of Witch Milk*? Well if you are not a medical student and you have heard it then you are really very well read. But for those who have not come across this bizarre phenomenon, let me explain.

Witch milk is the milk secreted from the nipples of infant on pinching them. Yes, you read it right. In newborn irrespective of male or female, this phenomenon can occur. Is there any explanation for this weird occurrence?

It is the mother's hormones that is still flowing in blood of infant, causing transient stimulation of lactational glands of the breast of infant. Activation of this gland can result in this phenomenon.

Let us pay close attention to what nature wants to convey. It says a lot many things, if we lend our ears. Male and female both are able to respond to female type of hormones. But in males this hormonal surge is suppressed. 'Y' chromosome is the reason, obviously.

During first year of my medical course, *human physiology* was one of the subjects. The physiology books used to be smaller and subject was quite easy as compared to other subjects. But I remember one exceptionally big book by *Best and Taylor.* It was so heavy and thick that it was difficult to carry.

Not many students dared to venture into this book. While browsing this voluminous giant of a book, I came across things that shook me up.

It has clearly mentioned, 'if a newborn male's nipples are continuously stimulated, that can bring out the female type of breast around puberty. I am not aware whether new edition of the book mentions it.

What is the conclusion? 'Y' chromosome has tried its best to suppress the hormonal surge. But continuous stimulation can rejuvenate that surge and cause female type of breast, which will not look so beautiful in a male body.

If you are not convinced still, I have got more facts to tell you. Here is the final blow.

There is something known as *gynecomastia*. What is gynecomastia? It is a female type of breast that is developed in the male body.

Can you tell me commonest age group in which it occurs? Yeah, you guessed it right. It is at the pubertal age. It occurs in some males at puberty. Obviously the 'Y' chromosome is still sleeping when the hormonal surge is occurring.

The strange thing about it is that, it is called *physiological*. If it occurs at puberty, it can be called Physiological, hmmm.............. that means it is natural. Can you believe it?

Are you thinking about the treatment for the same? Even if you are not, it is my duty to tell you as I have started this topic and pulled you into this. The treatment is wait and watch. As the boy surpasses his pubertal age, the gynecomastia gets corrected. It goes as smoothly as it had appeared. It disappears when the male crosses his puberty after giving him and his parents some anxious moments. It is a miracle. A male breast poses as female type for a while and then again turns flat.

What must have happened internally? It is anybody's guess. The sleeping 'Y' chromosome got awakened and though late, performed his duties.

Once again let's summarize what we have covered until now,

- At step I male had flat chest

- At step II male had female type of chest

- At step III male got back male type of chest

Let's corroborate it into chromosomal language.

'X' chromosome decides to have a female type of breast and has its way. But the 'Y' chromosome intervenes. Puts his foot forward and says 'no'. A strong 'no'! And in spite of that 'X' chromosome is adamant and produces the female type of breast, to announce its independence. 'Y' chromosome suppresses this mutiny with power. I want the flat chest, is the motto. 'Y' wins in the end.

This may be difficult to accept, I am aware. Something inside says, it shouldn't be like this. But the facts are there to be seen, discussed and debated.

We have observed that in almost all pubertal boys there is an insignificant type of pubertal development of gynecomastia. Only in some it becomes significant.

Before concluding this part of beautiful anatomy, let me tell you one more fact.

In the old age when 'Y' loses its vigor, there is a definite gynecomastia in most of the old men at around 70 to 80 years of age. Our bible, Surgical book of Love and Belly, depicts a beautiful picture of the old man with gynecomastia. To make matters worse in old age, gynecomastia is not reversible.

PART-III
Internal Beauty

Internal Genital Organs

Let's first finish the mechanical job of enumeration. Let's itemize the important organs of the internal genital system.

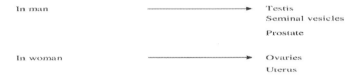

In man ⟶ Testis
Seminal vesicles
Prostate

In woman ⟶ Ovaries
Uterus

In male, all genital organs are opening outside through one common opening on the penis. Urethra also opens along with them.

Though far away from the topic, I cannot avoid the temptation of a doctor to mention it. In reality, urination and ejaculation cannot occur simultaneously. As both share a common opening, one system has to hold when other is venting.

The internal genital organs in female open into the vagina.

Let's peep into the animal world again. We have already talked about alligators. In alligators and in some frogs, male and female gender is not decided at birth. All eggs are same when they are laid. A male and female outcome is decided totally by the environmental factors. The most important factor is the temperature. Some scientists think humidity is also important.

At particular time and temperature, all eggs hatch to be males and at another but particular temperature all eggs hatch to be females.

Why is it important? I will soon elaborate. Until then, keep your brain warm, I mean keep this temperature factor always at the back of your mind.

Allow me to bombard your mind with more information over here. In a man, by that I mean male counterpart of human species; the abdominal temperature is always higher as compared to the scrotal temperature.

Nature has provided through the network of blood vessels, a special temperature control system to males. Why is this special arrangement? Which king resides in this scrotal palace? It's testicle.

At this juncture, the point to be noted is that the testicles change their character at different temperatures. At higher temperature they become sterile.

We have already talked about *hot furnace syndrome*. It is related to men constantly exposed to higher temperature.

The testicles at higher temperature undergo atrophy. They become sterile. Masculinity is lost. Only gun remains but no bullets. Seminal fluid stays without the sperms.

If this temperature exposure crosses a particular time limit, then changes become irreversible.

Extending the logic backwards - if heat is an important factor latter in life, can it be important in prenatal life? Do you remember the Chinese calendar?

Let's start with internal sexual organ counterparts in female and male - ovaries and testicles respectively. Initially we will consider the similarities. They both are round or spherical. They produce ova and sperms respectively which unite to form zygote.

In prenatal life they are both called primordial organs. Unbelievably, they both reside at the same level, at around the level of kidneys in the abdomen. That's upper most part of abdomen. They are almost identical in this aspect.

The great descent starts as the pregnancy progresses. Slowly but steadily they descend down in the abdomen in linear fashion. As pregnancy proceeds so does this, all important fall of organs.

When they reach up to the bladder, that would be lower compartment of abdomen, some significant changes occur in both of them. In females it is now full grown set of two ovaries.

In male it has to descend even more. The testicles descend to the level of bladder and then descend even more till they reach the scrotum and are thrown out of abdomen. Here they lock themselves into the scrotum.

What causes this great fall? Many believe it's the doing of the hormones. But I believe, although I have no proof, it must be temperature. Ligaments binding both these organs are not tight enough to hold their weight. Hence the great downfall occurs. The hormones even if they could be the cause, must be orchestrating these changes through temperature.

The ligaments are more elastic at higher temperature. So if temperature is higher the primordial organs fall even more to become testicles. As discussed earlier, the testicles have to be immediately cooled off to maintain their maleness. Thus heat is helpful in a way for masculinity but overheating could be disastrous.

Testicles cool off in scrotum to become their true self, whereas the primordial organs at the level of bladder constantly exposed to optimal abdominal temperature develop into ovaries.

To summarize,

	Woman	Man
Upper abdomen	Primordial organ	Primordial organ
Mid abdomen	Ovaries	Ovaries (Hypothetical)
Scrotum	—	Testis

There is another phenomenon called *undescended testis*. In this, testicles hang in between ovarian location and scrotum. The downfall occurs but is not sufficient. Primordial organs leave upper compartment of abdomen. They surpass ovarian location but do not reach scrotum. This is dangerous as heat can sterilize them. They have to be brought down by certain treatment, mainly by hormonal manipulation or by surgery. Of this hormonal treatment is almost a failure. And surgery is successful only if performed till a certain age. If they are not brought down in time, they undergo atrophy.

What does it indicate? The ovaries and testicles are basically same. But one is exposed to certain temperature for a particular period to grow into ovaries. Whereas testicles are cooled within time to maintain their integrity.

Can this conclusion be drawn? I leave it to you.

Another important thing to remember is unless testicles come down to scrotum, the scrotal development does not occur. Hence the emperor testis decides the development of scrotum. Until the weight of the testis acts, the scrotum remains flat just like labia majora in females. This fact can help in visualization of the fusion of labia in females as described above.

This concludes the discussion on most important factors that decide the gender – male or female.

In next chapter we shall put the spotlight on accessory internal genital organs viz. prostate and seminal vesicles in male and uterus and fallopian tubes in female.

Accessory Internal Genital Organs

Let's start with the female organs. I will first discuss the uterus and uterine tubes and it's relation to ovaries.

Have you seen the movie, *'Sleepy Hollow'*? Do you remember the headless horseman looking for his own head? Then you should look at the drawing given below and use your imagination.

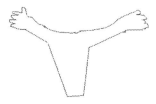

Does it look like a headless man stretching arms to reach up to the ovaries? The uterus along with fallopian tubes will look like this.

This whole structure lies between rectum (that is terminal part of intestines) and bladder, in a pouch called recto-uterine pouch. It is much easier over here. If one goes down towards end of the bladder, the space gets congested. So it can afford to stretch its arms over here but not further down. Essentially we are discussing female organ here, but as per our conclusion it has to get converted into male part if the fall continues.

If the ovaries can fall below to become the testicles, can these accessories remain behind? The emperor has gone down to the scrotal place, so the body guards have to follow!

Let us keep things simple. Let us imagine a bit. Once again, awaken the Steven Spielberg that resides within you.

What happens if this structure goes below the bladder level?

There the space is congested and as a result the movement is restricted and one has to fight for his space. Below the bladder lies urethra. Therefore the headless man has to fold his arms and engulf the relatively tubular structure of the urethra.

The bladder is more like a bag as compared to urethra.

So it looks somewhat like this

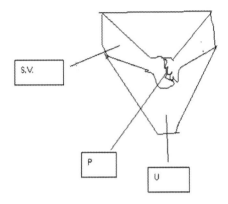

S.V.   Seminal vesicle

U.   Urethra

P.   Prostate

Do you see the picture? This is exactly how male accessory sexual organs are arranged.

The discussion until now makes it clear that

- A person cannot be differentiated as male or female in the beginning

- Then a phase with dominant female characters occurs

- Some halt at this stage and enjoy being females for the rest of their life

- Others mature into male

To summarize

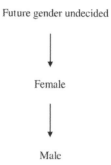

Future gender undecided

Female

Male

To put it into scientific language, all humans are females to start with. Some develop further to become males.

Scrotal Development and Some Clues

This is supposed to be a short chapter. Though short, it is very important for our hypothesis. It might change the course of sex change operations in future.

We have seen that scrotal development in true sense does not begin till the testicular descent is complete. As a matter of fact - the hormones secreted from testis and its weight contributes significantly to scrotal development. Then there is another fact. In patients with testis that has not descended, scrotum never develops.

What do we mean by scrotal development? In the beginning scrotal skin is very flat. The creases, mark of adult scrotum, are absent. In fact it is just like the vulval skin without the cleft, as discussed earlier. To be more precise instead of cleft there is a prominent joint mark as if someone has stitched the cleft completely.

As the testicles come and reside inside scrotum, the growth of scrotal skin speeds up. It exceeds the speed of development of skin over rest of the body. As the cover is always bigger than the content, the scrotal skin has to get partially folded in order to fit over the scrotum and that's the reason behind the creases. As the skin increases in length so does the underlying blood vessels. This serves the purpose of cooling the testicles to keep them firm and functional.

Apart from this development, there is not much difference between scrotum and vulva.

As far as the contents are concerned the testicles reside in scrotum in male. In female, ovaries are in abdomen hence vulva is empty.

Scrotum in general is improvised vulva. This helps to prove our hypothesis. Man is an extension of woman. Scrotum presents itself as the external manifestation of the internal series of changes that has to take place inside woman in order to get converted into man.

PART-IV
Emotions and
Intelligence

Behavioral Patterns

Psychologically, and in some way intellectually, women are different than men. Social behavior of any individual depends upon these two factors – psychological and intellectual.

Let's consider behavioral differences. Behavioral difference between two is very evident in dress code. Just looking at a dress, one can conclude if the person is male or female. Considering the physical differences, it is natural. Dress code in different societies is different for women. But the aim seems to be to dress up a woman in such a manner so as not to arouse man's desire.

The social norms of the locality also play their role. However, in advanced countries it seems that these sensitivities are not stringently followed.

The ability to control the surroundings (climate control, artificial rains etc.) to some extent and the freedom issues of the woman also play their role

In societies where the dominant opinion abhors provocative dresses, the dress code of women is quite different from the men whereas in liberal societies a woman can wear clothes like man i.e. trousers and shirts.

In the field of entertainment, woman's dress code is rather modern but in line with the requirements of the industry that they operate in. In medical profession, male as well as female nurses and doctors have similar dresses but they are distinctly different than the way engineers dress up at their sites. Thus a dress code has more to do with career rather than being a male or a female unless one gets bogged down by the social pressure in closely knit communities.

In short it can be said that in more progressive society, woman is trying to achieve a relaxed outfit like man and in that sense her progression towards being a man has actually began. It is easy to discard this argument and look at it more as demands of job. But looking around, it is easy to spot females shedding clothing to look attractive, modern and appealing. This is not just due to the requirements of a job where women don't need to attract unwarranted attention. It is rather a case of projecting oneself – confident, dominant and professional – qualities that have traditionally defined a male.

One very important observation needs to be mentioned over here. When a woman tries to upgrade her dress code and tries to appear like a male, it could be considered normal in progressive society. However when man tries to do similar thing and dresses like a female, it is not appreciated that much. Does it ring a bell? Can it prove a point over here? Yes. Obviously if you progress (towards manhood) it is considered normal but if you regress towards womanhood, how could it be normal?

This concludes our discussion on dress code.

The way woman walks or talks or sits also differs from a man. But most of it is determined by the way you dress up. If you wear a skirt, you have to sit cross legged. If you wear high heel foot wares, you will walk differently. Walking, talking and sitting of woman are changing for sure. A woman is getting closer in behavior to a man.

The other behavioral changes are more to confirm to social norms. We as a society have decided certain guidelines for woman to behave in public. Along with society the guidelines are changing too.

Not only for woman but also for man with different jobs, castes, or race, there are certain subtle guidelines. If we think about it we can see it more clearly.

Have you observed how a doctor talks and how a police man talks? How a military man is disciplined and how an artist can spend time in bed till noon?

We as a society have decided a certain code of conduct for everybody depending upon what he or she does. If you see them behave differently, a social reaction is aroused depending upon how tolerant the society is.

These social norms are not limited to careers alone. Inside our minds we have formed views on how people from different countries would behave. Many acceptable things in America suddenly become unacceptable when the American goes to Afghanistan. Over here, the same American will change his code of conduct to a considerable extent. Vice versa is also true.

A woman does not behave in a particular manner by nature but the society dictates her to behave in a certain way. Otherwise how does one explain the changes as they locate to new places and grow in age? They even behave differently with different people. A daughter in law in India will behave entirely different in front of her father than in front of her father in law.

In Saudi Arabia, country known for its restrictive traditions for the fairer sex – women are not allowed to drive, they cannot step out of their homes without a male escort who has to be a close relative – women party and although alcoholic drink that is banned is not served, women are known to smoke heavily.

In developed society where a woman has emancipated to work shoulder to shoulder with man, the prominent differences in clothing, smoking, drinking, partying, betting, travelling etc. are fast disappearing. Look at the women in police or military and you will appreciate the change. And if you hear them shout the way men do, lingering doubts over their delicate nature will disappear in thin air.

Women are overwhelmed by the patriarchal laws that govern their behavior in public. Given a choice, they would be as liberal as men.

Men, on the other hand, enjoy freedom of choice. They are mostly unrestricted. Yet, you will not find them imitating women.

What's the point of this discussion?

It is difficult for a man to behave like a woman and if he does, it is considered abnormal. In case of a woman, it is much easier to adopt a man's life style. In progressive societies, this natural process has already taken root.

Emotions and Intelligence

Irishmen in English, Sardars in India, blondes in America and women universally share the same spot. They are at the centre of jokes. Their supposed fickle mindedness boosts creativity in other people. They have been at the receiving end of humor for ages.

'Behind every successful man is a woman' – the famous quote associates success with a man and sacrifice to a woman behind him. Why is woman always behind?

Man is considered to be intellectually superior to woman. The origin of this belief is not very clear. But constant devotion of female to her family (in fact the word *family* is quiet closer to the word *female*) her submission, her sacrifice of career for the sake of children etc. are considered affectionate but worldly not so wise. At times, they have been labeled '*emotional fools*', meaning thereby, to succumb to their emotions.

There are certain concerns regarding the intelligence of females. How many females are known as great chess players or how many women lead their nation as heads of state? I beg to differ from this kind of mind set. I think the situation points more towards lack of opportunities for women than anything else.

Let us consider a game of chess; it is known that the best chess players are from Russia. Does that make people from rest of the world including Americans, Japanese, Indians or Chinese, intellectually inferior to Russians?

In Russia it is a nationwide passion, so environment is conducive to produce world class chess players. What is true for Russians in Chess is true for Americans in cars or Chinese in hardware or Indians in software.

Rather than deliberating further on how many great women chess players are active in the world, it would be interesting to find out number of females who start the game at an early age and how many of them are encouraged by society.

As for heading the nation is considered, I think it is more by chance than design that the person is chosen. The human psychological evolution is not complete. But as a proud Indian I know Mrs. Indira Gandhi had headed India remarkably well during her tenure.

While discussing the nonsexual internal organ, I had not touched upon brain in detail. The brain in females is on an average smaller in size. Does that make her less intelligent? Japanese brain may be on an average smaller in size as compared to European. Does that make European more intelligent?

Let's revisit the Animal Kingdom. What about elephants or dolphins? Are they superior to humans? Was Dinosaur more intelligent than most known animals? Who is intellectually more evolved cannot be determined by the size of the brain alone.

It is a proven fact that the ratio of body mass to brain mass, determines the intelligence. Let us extend our hypothesis to the situation on hand. I think the routine and complex procedures performed by the body consume a lot of brain's attention. So if an elephant has to constantly eat with his trunk, the brain is monitoring the process closely and very less time is available to develop intelligence for other things. Why people meditate is, to somehow increase this intelligence for creative purpose rather than wasting it on routine.

Let's stop here as it is not subject of our discussion but not without the food for imagination. Does this brain body mass index mean, if a person reduces his weight, he will become more intelligent?

Emotional behavior of man and woman is distinct. They are definitely different on an emotional plane. Let me develop some background before I pull you into the vortex of something that is slightly more complex.

Man	Woman
Reserved	More open
Aggressive	Docile
Tears are unknown	Tears flow like rain
Apathetic	Sympathetic
Dominative	Submissive
Impulsive	Thoughtful
Rough & tough	Caring
Driven by physique (physical skill, Strength)	Use of soft skills (talking, empathizing)

Let's catalog emotional differences between man and woman.

Keep this knowledge at the back of your mind. We shall use it soon. First, we need to differentiate between what we feel and how we express it.

A particular man may be tremendously happy yet keep his face sober whereas somebody else may demonstrate his joy by jumping in air. One look at the final of any sport would explain the point. Many of us born in 60's and 70's would definitely recall the icy Bjohn Borg and feisty John McEnroe playing in the final of Wimbledon Lawn Tennis Competition or the cricket loving world will never forget India's first World Cup win in 1983 when the leading bowler of defending Champions West Indies, Malcom Marshall cried inconsolably.

Have you attended a funeral? Plethora of human expressions can be witnessed there. Some people cry, some shout with grief, some curse the God. There are also people who remain calm and silent. Does that mean they are not affected?

Thus a strong distinction has to be made between what we feel and how we express that feeling. A woman is in summary more expressive. But what's felt or how it is felt inside may not be very different.

This point forms an important cornerstone of our further discussion as such I hope I have made it abundantly clear.

For simplicity, let us divide people into two categories - expressive and non-expressive. Usually non-expressive people can start to express themselves with an outside stimulus. This can be in the form of a motivational speech, inspirational movie or an alcoholic drink.

Let the non-expressive men drink and observe the change in them. They will shout, cry, laugh, jump or do crazy things to vent out their inner feelings. The dose of alcohol will vary from person to person but the important thing here is a non-expressive person will start to express himself.

What does it mean to us?

If we consider the emotional outburst to be the right of woman then it will give us a strange reality.

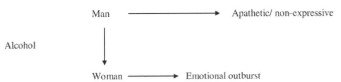

A man is still the man; only the way of expression of his feeling is changed. What acts like alcohol in day to day life? Do women drink a lot clandestinely? Obviously, the answer to that is no. Hormones make woman more sensitive to a situation than man. During a period of hormonal outburst in her body, woman prefers to be left alone. This is physiological and is referred as 'menstrual psychosis'.

Let us move further now that we have established why a woman is emotionally different from a man. She is definitely different and that is accepted. I want to raise another question at this juncture – has the woman changed over passage of time?

Look at the emotional development of woman over the generations. This task is made easier by comparison of old classics with modern movies. Can you say the emotional outburst of a woman has remained same over a period? A cursory glance at emotional scenes in movies of different era will clarify the matter.

Woman is becoming less expressive with the passage of time. Does that mean she is competing with a man and losing her power of empathy?

Are emotionally men and women moving towards each other?

Thank goodness, woman continues to be more sensitive than a man, at least till now. However, there is a question mark dangling over humanity if she is as sensitive as a woman of around hundred years ago. We can attribute many reasons to change of attitude and we can all agree over them – change of life style, working at office as well as handing responsibilities at home, career mindedness etc.

There are indications that the menopause among women has started to happen early – is the nature fastening process of evolution of woman to a man? Another recent observation is that the menstruation among women has also advanced. As recent as 1950s, on an average, girls at the age of 15 used to enter puberty but now the recent study suggests that this process starts at 13 – reduction of 2 years in 5 decades is a cause for worry.

Hundred years from now, will the woman still maintain her level of empathy? Will the difference be more noticeable over thousand years? Humans will have to wait and see. Let's conclude our third part here and move on to something more interesting.

PART - V
Master of the Game
and the Cycle of Life

The Master Manipulator

Chemical intervention in human body has gone beyond our imagination. Sometimes, we can see the external manifestations of this process by naked eyes. But for these chemical reactions to be detected, one needs the help of sophisticated laboratories. The drugs and even food can induce some chemical reaction inside of human body. They are introduced from outside. But there is something of its own, that is acting from inside.

Consider the growth of human body from childhood to death. Look at it as a movie. Externally the body grows from childhood to adulthood. Then as the old age approaches, deterioration begins. Many body parts slowly lose their capacity to function normally. Ultimately the death occurs.

What happens internally within a body during these changes? How much effort is taken to keep that movie smooth and pleasant to eyes goes unrecognized.

The directors of this movie are chemical substances called hormones. However, the producer of the movie is a matter of faith.

By definition, a hormone is any substance, which is, produced at one place in a body (glands) and spreads through the blood, to affect almost all the reactions in the body in some or the other way.

Modus operandi is almost the same for all hormones.

There is a stimulus. This may be external or internal, physical or chemical or sometimes even visual. Upon stimulation a kind of chemical trigger is pulled. Depending upon type of stimulus, a specific hormone will start getting secreted. This secretion of hormone can itself pull other triggers, to start other hormones getting secreted. But that cycle is more complex and is not required to prove our point. Hence I will concentrate upon the first stimulus and the hormone secreted.

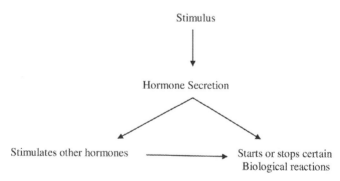

Through the blood the hormone is taken to its work place which may be entirely different part of body than the place of its origin. Body reacts to these secretions.

If it is in growing phase, it shows growth in certain direction or regression in other directions.

Hormone continues to get secreted or stops. In first case hormone continues to modify physical as well as psychological outcomes. In the second case the direction for future bodily changes is predetermined.

There are certain hormones in the body, which are common in male and female. So they bring about the same physical and if at all psychological outcomes in both.

In early years of life they bring about growth and in later years they maintain metabolism. Thyroxin, growth hormones, cortisones are some of the hormones from this category. In their absence, a particular disease is formed which is also common in male and female.

As far as common hormones in both the sexes are concerned, they will cause similar reactions in both male as well as female. But are we interested in them? They don't serve any purpose to the topic of this book.

Let's now turn our attention to sex hormones and learn interesting facts about them. They differentiate emotional, psychological and physical make up of male and female.

Our interest is in two hormones, estrogen (E) and testosterone (T). E is feminine and T is masculine.

They both act on human body. Let's call it H. Action of E and T on H produces drastically different results.

They convert H into psychophysical complexes named female and male.

A pubertal boy with gynecomastia is not a girl. But he is referred to as a boy with physiological gynecomastia.

The hormone is a master of the game. But sometimes it gets confused because E and T are inter-convertible. Estrogen can be converted into testosterone and by some chemical metabolic process T loses part of its molecular structure to become E.

In old age this is the cause of gynecomastia and even in pubertal gynecomastia which is fascinatingly called physiological, estrogen surge is the reason.

Let me hypothetically extend this inter-convertibility factor.

E = T-1 or 2 or any no.

Or otherwise T= E+1, 2, or any no.

It can also be E = T / 2 or T = 2E or 3 E or something like that.

To understand its implication, it is better to know psychological and physical effects of E and T.

Psychologically speaking, E induces sensitivity and T causes aggressiveness. E is submissive and shy, T is dominant and violent. Physically, T extends or pulls or modifies certain bodily parts except for breasts. Breasts are typically suppressed by T.

The effects of E and T ware off. They exit from the body. However, their exit from the body takes a lot of time. Almost a lifetime! I said almost not entire life time.

- At menopause, a woman loses all of her E.

- At the same time in man, most of the T produced is getting converted into E.

How will you describe these events? A male is getting converted into a female?

A woman may tell a lot about how difficult it is to be a woman in this harsh world. But yet if we offer her the sex change operation, chances are she might refuse. So we always like to be what we are in spite of few disadvantages. We cling to our identity as a man or a woman.

In general, woman loves to be a woman. But little does she know that all her womanhood depends upon E and its production. The woman becomes old. At this stage, the Estrogen storage reduces as the production stops and the consumption is high. This is an interesting case. Something called *postmenopausal syndrome* occurs.

It is filled with agitation, irritation and inexplicable feeling of restlessness. Many ladies face the identity crisis in this situation.

Physically she starts losing her hair on scalp. Some women develop beards. The definite contour of breasts is lost. So in general, she is losing her womanhood. At a subconscious level she is aware of this fact and that produces restlessness. These changes are killing her. Some women lose their psyche up to the level of madness! This is all a result of lack of production of the estrogen by the body.

Can you think of any treatment for this weird phenomenon? You guessed it right; it is called *'HRT or Hormone Replacement Therapy'*. Ultimately it is E supplementation.

Many people think that men don't have menopauses. Many orthodox people will use this point to underline the fact that man is superior.

Man does not have a definite point where the menopause occurs. He may not show definite sign like menopause in females where she stops menstruating.

In old age many men develop gynecomastia. Some develop loss of libido or sexual desire. Some men suddenly develop phenomenon of losing affinity towards life. Some manifest strange phenomenon of increased libido. I will call it a cry of dying masculinity. It is self-limiting. May be it is a last try of T to utilize its vanishing resources which is so closely linked with manhood. Hence the menopause is occurring but it is gradual and subtle.

Here is what we have discussed so for,

- Man or woman is born

- At puberty fully grown man or woman develops

- At menopause E or T resources are finished

- Physical changes towards opposite gender, start appearing

The death occurs at this particular juncture. What if death is delayed by a considerable time? To what extent these changes will take place?

The conclusion of this entire chapter depends upon only one person and that's you. I will leave you with the thought that, what if the man and woman continue to live beyond their menopause, for another life time?

The Cycle of Life

Do you believe in theory of *'Karma'?* Birth, death and rebirth are three aspects of this theory. According to this theory life revolves in cycles.

In Hindu scriptures a stage of *'Moksha'* is described. This is the permanent release of soul, breaking free from phenomenon of birth and death.

Everything in world revolves in a cycle. Life revolves in cycle and the Moksha is breaking away from this cycle.

There is an epic called *Mahabharata*. It describes the Great War that occurred in ancient India many centuries ago. In this war some classic weapons were used. There was a weapon which could be used by a selected few, called *'Brahmastra'*. Astra mean weapon and Brahmastra means the ultimate weapon. It could be fired from a bow. The devastating effects of Brahmastra are described vividly. It is equivalent to modern day atomic bomb explosion.

Now why sudden diversion from the discussion of the genetics, man and woman to atomic bomb?

You must be startled. I don't blame you.

Consider two cycles simultaneously taking place in the universe. One cycle is small and other is very big.

In a smaller cycle a man dies and is reborn, dies again and the cycle continues.

In a bigger cycle, through the amino acid production (the building blocks of life in general) smaller life forms like amoeba are coming to existence. Amoeba is a single cell animal. The single cell animals unite to form more complex animals. Then bigger animals are formed and then the ultimate big dinosaurs come into existence.

Meanwhile, somewhere else a monkey is changing into something intelligent. *Homo sapiens* announce its arrival.

At first he is controlled by the nature. Then by using his brain, he discovers some tools which can be used as weapons. Then he starts killing the animals which could trouble him sometimes.

The aim until now was the survival of the species. He discovers more weapons along the way. He kills some animals and tames some. He starts to control nature.

There is no threat to his species now. He has to find another aim. He forms groups within human species.

They continue to discover new weapons to achieve dominance among themselves.

Ultimately weapons of mass destruction come to existence and boom!

Everything is destroyed. The earth is lifeless.

After many unrecorded centuries amino acid is produced at the sea shore. The bigger cycle continues!

There is an equation of mass and energy. The product of energy and mass is constant, although they are inter-convertible. Life in true sense is energy. Consider this as the equation of mass and life. At any point on earth the product of life and mass has to remain constant.

Someone has written the fate of the man as he was born, he suffered and he died. Very pessimistic view! I strongly disagree with this. Fate is the end point. End point has to be present on the linear path. But if pathway is twisted into circle, there won't be any starting or end point. It will just revolve around itself. Every starting point could as well be an end point.

We all know that energy flows into circles. Similarly life flows into circles because life is equivalent to energy. Individual man comes and goes, life remains. In nature everything flows in a circle.

Open any biological book, you will find many cycles of biological process that occur inside the body. There is description of even the life cycles of bacteria and the fungi.

Open any biochemistry book; there will be description of cycles of biochemical processes, occurring inside the body of a living thing.

There is one beautiful poem. My uncle used to recite it for me, in my childhood. It was in *Marathi*, my mother tongue. It read like this, there was a droplet of water lying in the river bed, playing and enjoying its life. As it was winter, the droplet was cold, but not too cold to flow, to jump and to mix with the other droplets.

But soon winter got over and hot summer started. It made the sun shine brighter. It became intolerable now. The droplet got angry. It started fuming. The anger got better of him and he got converted into a vapor.

It could fly. It left the mother river. It flied up, up and above. There was sadness of departure, but joy of achievement. It was a mixed feeling. The droplet would fly as it could, but in the wee hours, it would become tired and heavy. It would again come down and settle upon rose petal and sleep there as dewdrop.

It would sleep till the sun came up and evaporate again to fly up. It continued for a while till the droplet was bored. The droplet was bored to be alone. The droplet wanted a company.

So it flew up, up and above, suddenly he found many droplets flowing together. It was a big black cloud. The droplet joined them. They floated together like expert gliders from tree tops to mountains to empty sky. It was fun.

One day they were floating above the river. Monsoon was around the corner. Seeing the river, the cloud rained upon it. The droplet came down as raindrop. It was again flowing with the river.

All the time, the droplet wondered about its origin.

You can easily see that the poem ended at the same point where it had started.

Amazingly, it could start at any point provided it ends at the same point.

So the droplet could be a part of cloud and ultimately mix with cloud. It could start on rose petal as dewdrop and end there as dewdrop.

All the while droplet could wonder where it has come from. Because droplet could not understand that it is life which is running in circle.

So our life also runs in circle. We start at birth and then from infancy, we become young. Then a full grown woman or man is developed.

Over here, one life time is consumed. The menopause is reached towards the end of the life. At this juncture man or woman is getting converted into opposite sex. Before the changes are too prominent to be ignored, the man or woman is dead. They go to the grave with the secret.

But what if we live long enough to see further changes in one life time only?

That is the big question I guess! I am concluding my book over here as I have nothing more to say on this topic. It may seem to end abruptly but your imagination power will fill up the lacunae. I am sure about that.

There is no such thing as,   THE END

Glossary

A

Abdomen L. *abdere* to hide

Anatomy Gr. *ana* apart, *tome* to cut

Axilla L. armpit

C

Cervix L. neck

Chromosome L.*chroma* colour, *soma* body

Clitoris Gr. *kleitoris* from *kleiein* to shut up

E

Embryo Gr. *en* in *bryein* to swell

F

Fetus L. offspring

H

Hormone Gr. *hormaein* to excite

L

Labium L. a lip *labia* plu.

Lactation *lactis* milk

Lacuna L. a pit

O

Ovum L. an egg

P

Penis L. a tail

Prostate Gr. *pro* before, *histanai* to set ,one who stands before

R

Rectum L. straight

S

Scrotum L. a bag

Sperm Gr. *sperma* a seed

Syndrome Gr. *syn* with, *dramein* to run

T

Testis L. a witness(of sex, hence male gonad)

U

Ureter Gr. *oureter* urinary canal

Urethra Gr. *ourethra* urethra

Uterus L. womb

V

Vagina L. a sheath

Viscera L. from *viscus,* an internal organ

Vulva L. a wrapper, from *volvere* to roll

Z

Zygote Gr. from *zygon* a yoke